How to stop hair loss -
1: Don't get married!
2: Don't have children!

**How to stop hair loss -
1: Don't get married!
2: Don't have children!**

How To Stop Hair Loss

Written By Terry Billitch
Cover photograph by Ocusfocus
Copyright Argle Bargle Publishing Ltd

Foreword and Disclaimer.

**This book is a novelty joke book and not
intended as a serious guide,
we suggest using it as a notepad.**

**The Author and Publisher take no responsibility
for any advice contained within the book.
This book is purely for entertainment purposes only and
should not be viewed as a genuine way of solving
hair loss issues.**

**How to stop hair loss -
1: Don't get married!
2: Don't have children!**

How to stop hair loss -
1: Don't get married!
2: Don't have children!

How to stop hair loss -
1: Don't get married!
2: Don't have children!

How to stop hair loss -
1: Don't get married!
2: Don't have children!

How to stop hair loss -
1: Don't get married!
2: Don't have children!

**How to stop hair loss -
1: Don't get married!
2: Don't have children!**

**How to stop hair loss -
1: Don't get married!
2: Don't have children!**

**How to stop hair loss -
1: Don't get married!
2: Don't have children!**

**How to stop hair loss -
1: Don't get married!
2: Don't have children!**

**How to stop hair loss -
1: Don't get married!
2: Don't have children!**

How to stop hair loss -
1: Don't get married!
2: Don't have children!

**How to stop hair loss -
1: Don't get married!
2: Don't have children!**

**How to stop hair loss -
1: Don't get married!
2: Don't have children!**

How to stop hair loss -
1: Don't get married!
2: Don't have children!

**How to stop hair loss -
1: Don't get married!
2: Don't have children!**

**How to stop hair loss -
1: Don't get married!
2: Don't have children!**

How to stop hair loss -
1: Don't get married!
2: Don't have children!

**How to stop hair loss -
1: Don't get married!
2: Don't have children!**

**How to stop hair loss -
1: Don't get married!
2: Don't have children!**

**How to stop hair loss -
1: Don't get married!
2: Don't have children!**

**How to stop hair loss -
1: Don't get married!
2: Don't have children!**

How to stop hair loss -
1: Don't get married!
2: Don't have children!

How to stop hair loss -
1: Don't get married!
2: Don't have children!

**How to stop hair loss -
1: Don't get married!
2: Don't have children!**

How to stop hair loss -
1: Don't get married!
2: Don't have children!

**How to stop hair loss -
1: Don't get married!
2: Don't have children!**

How to stop hair loss -
1: Don't get married!
2: Don't have children!

**How to stop hair loss -
1: Don't get married!
2: Don't have children!**

How to stop hair loss -
1: Don't get married!
2: Don't have children!

How to stop hair loss -
1: Don't get married!
2: Don't have children!

How to stop hair loss -
1: Don't get married!
2: Don't have children!

**How to stop hair loss -
1: Don't get married!
2: Don't have children!**

**How to stop hair loss -
1: Don't get married!
2: Don't have children!**

**How to stop hair loss -
1: Don't get married!
2: Don't have children!**

**How to stop hair loss -
1: Don't get married!
2: Don't have children!**

**How to stop hair loss -
1: Don't get married!
2: Don't have children!**

**How to stop hair loss -
1: Don't get married!
2: Don't have children!**

How to stop hair loss -
1: Don't get married!
2: Don't have children!

How to stop hair loss -
1: Don't get married!
2: Don't have children!

**How to stop hair loss -
1: Don't get married!
2: Don't have children!**

**How to stop hair loss -
1: Don't get married!
2: Don't have children!**

**How to stop hair loss -
1: Don't get married!
2: Don't have children!**

**How to stop hair loss -
1: Don't get married!
2: Don't have children!**

**How to stop hair loss -
1: Don't get married!
2: Don't have children!**

**How to stop hair loss -
1: Don't get married!
2: Don't have children!**

**How to stop hair loss -
1: Don't get married!
2: Don't have children!**

How to stop hair loss -
1: Don't get married!
2: Don't have children!

**How to stop hair loss -
1: Don't get married!
2: Don't have children!**

**How to stop hair loss -
1: Don't get married!
2: Don't have children!**

**How to stop hair loss -
1: Don't get married!
2: Don't have children!**

**How to stop hair loss -
1: Don't get married!
2: Don't have children!**

How to stop hair loss -
1: Don't get married!
2: Don't have children!

How to stop hair loss -
1: Don't get married!
2: Don't have children!

**How to stop hair loss -
1: Don't get married!
2: Don't have children!**

How to stop hair loss -
1: Don't get married!
2: Don't have children!

**How to stop hair loss -
1: Don't get married!
2: Don't have children!**

**How to stop hair loss -
1: Don't get married!
2: Don't have children!**

How to stop hair loss -
1: Don't get married!
2: Don't have children!

How to stop hair loss -
1: Don't get married!
2: Don't have children!

**How to stop hair loss -
1: Don't get married!
2: Don't have children!**

How to stop hair loss -
1: Don't get married!
2: Don't have children!

How to stop hair loss -
1: Don't get married!
2: Don't have children!

How to stop hair loss -
1: Don't get married!
2: Don't have children!

How to stop hair loss -
1: Don't get married!
2: Don't have children!

**How to stop hair loss -
1: Don't get married!
2: Don't have children!**

How to stop hair loss -
1: Don't get married!
2: Don't have children!

How to stop hair loss -
1: Don't get married!
2: Don't have children!

How to stop hair loss -
1: Don't get married!
2: Don't have children!

How to stop hair loss -
1: Don't get married!
2: Don't have children!

**How to stop hair loss -
1: Don't get married!
2: Don't have children!**

How to stop hair loss -
1: Don't get married!
2: Don't have children!

How to stop hair loss -
1: Don't get married!
2: Don't have children!

**How to stop hair loss -
1: Don't get married!
2: Don't have children!**

How to stop hair loss -
1: Don't get married!
2: Don't have children!

**How to stop hair loss -
1: Don't get married!
2: Don't have children!**

How to stop hair loss -
1: Don't get married!
2: Don't have children!

**How to stop hair loss -
1: Don't get married!
2: Don't have children!**

**How to stop hair loss -
1: Don't get married!
2: Don't have children!**

How to stop hair loss -
1: Don't get married!
2: Don't have children!

**How to stop hair loss -
1: Don't get married!
2: Don't have children!**

How to stop hair loss -
1: Don't get married!
2: Don't have children!

**How to stop hair loss -
1: Don't get married!
2: Don't have children!**

**How to stop hair loss -
1: Don't get married!
2: Don't have children!**